Remember, Dad?

Remember, Dad?

A Journey into Memory Loss

Lorlie Barkman

Winnipeg, Manitoba

KINDRED
PRODUCTIONS

Hillsboro, Kansas

Remember, Dad?

Published simultaneously by Kindred Productions, Winnipeg, Manitoba R2L 2E5 and
Kindred Productions, Hillsboro. Kansas 67063.

Printed by Hignell Book Printing

Canadian Cataloguing in Publication Data

Barkman, Lorlie 1941-
       Remember, Dad?
       ISBN: 0-921788-61-4
1. Art theory. 2. Caricatures and cartoons. 3. Memory disorders in old age. 4 Memory disorders–Patients–Rehabilitation. 5. Barkman family–Anecdotes. I.Title.

RC489.A7B27 1999   616.89' 1656   C99-920212-X

Special Thanks

———◆———

To my wife, Deanna, a nurse, for her patience and valuable insights; to my family and caregivers everywhere, and to Dora Dueck for her perceptions as an editor.

INTRODUCTION

When my father began to show signs of memory loss as he approached the age of 80, we in the family began a journey that would take us through new, and often puzzling and painful, experiences. Even as we struggled with our denial, a wise and caring community health care worker, understanding Dad's symptoms, pressed upon us the need to prepare for what lay ahead. She gave us an image to help us balance the loss coming upon us like shadows at twilight with the rest of Dad's life. Seeing our loved one gradually lose his memory and sense of reality, she said, was like watching drapes close slowly over a window. Look for the moments, she encouraged us further, no matter how fleeting, when the drapes would open temporarily, even just a crack, and let in a ray of light. That bit of advice brought us hope and goodness. It helped us discover that the image of God created in Dad continued to exist even when so much of what we had known of him seemed lost.

By the time my father entered a personal care home, it was becoming increasingly difficult to communicate with him by letter or telephone, particularly from a distance. I have a background in cartooning and have done some reading in art therapy. Because Dad's memory of the past was better than his awareness of the present, I came up with the idea of drawing cartoons of some of the events in his life, describing each picture briefly in a paragraph and sending them to him. Staff in the care home said he cherished the drawings and related well to them. Once he brought a drawing to the nursing station, saying, "Now it's my turn!" He proceeded to describe in detail how he fit into the picture.

Unfortunately, I was able to send him only three of these pictures before he died. On further reflection, it occurred to me that I could do a whole series of story illustrations to trace his journey through what was probably Alzheimer's disease, even if only for the family.

This was good therapy for me. It also became a valuable exercise in discovering that not all is lost, even in the tragedy of memory loss. Although it is hard to see a loved one in the shadows cast by failing light, there can still be moments of gratification. I say this recognizing that my father did not live for a prolonged time in the most severe conditions of Alzheimer's. Just the same, what I experienced has been helpful in my own ministry of caregiving.

David, the Psalm writer in the Bible, expressed the nature of his humanness before God in this way: "You created my inmost being; you knit me together in my mother's womb. I praise you because I am fearfully and wonderfully made; your works are wonderful, I know that full well" (Psalm 139:13-14). When losses like those brought on by Alzheimer's disease beset someone we know, we may think that all goodness will be lost. But something of the presence of God remains. We may have to look carefully to see it, but it is there.

In *The Return of the Prodigal*, Henri Nouwen writes:

> "People who have come to know the joy of God do not deny the darkness,
> but they choose not to live in it. They claim that the light that shines in
> the darkness can be trusted more than the darkness itself and that a
> little bit of light can dispel a lot of darkness. They point each other to
> flashes of light here and there, and remind each other that they reveal
> the hidden but real presence of God." (117)

This comforting truth, as we experienced it in my father's last years, is what these pictures and words celebrate.

Lorlie Barkman
August, 1999

Dear Dad:

You were born and raised in the little farming community called "Flowing Well." I remember hearing the story of how it got its name. In 1908, an elderly pioneer with white hair and whiskers built a shack and began to dig for water. He dug the first six feet himself. Then he had someone else go into the hole and dig while he hauled up the dirt with a rope and pail. When the hole was 26 feet deep, they heard the sound of running water. The digger climbed out with his spade and the two men went for lunch. When they came back, they were surprised to find the hole full of water. Not only full, but flowing over! I remember pulling up a pail of cold, crystal-clear water for a drink on a hot day. No water ever tasted as good as that coming from the flowing well.

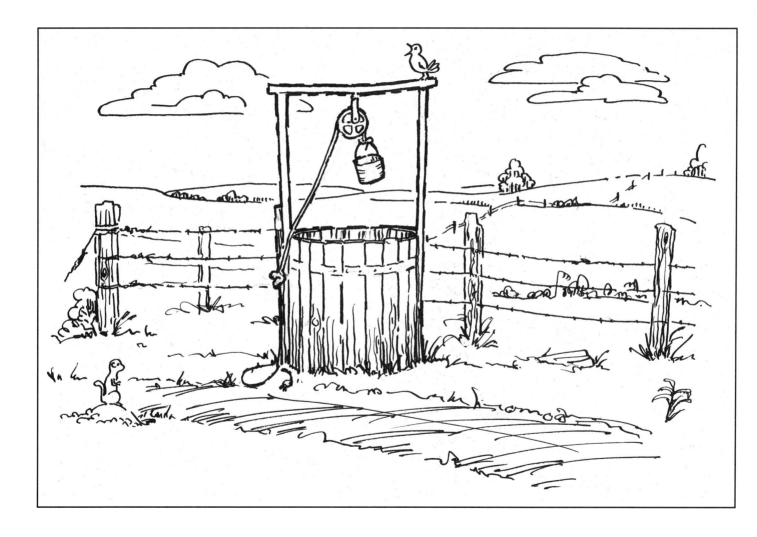

Dear Dad:

You had a tear in your voice whenever you told us the story of how your mother looked after you as a child, especially when you were sick. She would come to check on you at night, upstairs in the rambling old farmhouse. She lit a coal oil lamp and placed it beside your bed, letting it burn all night with the wick turned low. The only time she set the lamp out for you was when you were ill. Something about that experience made you emotional every time you told it.

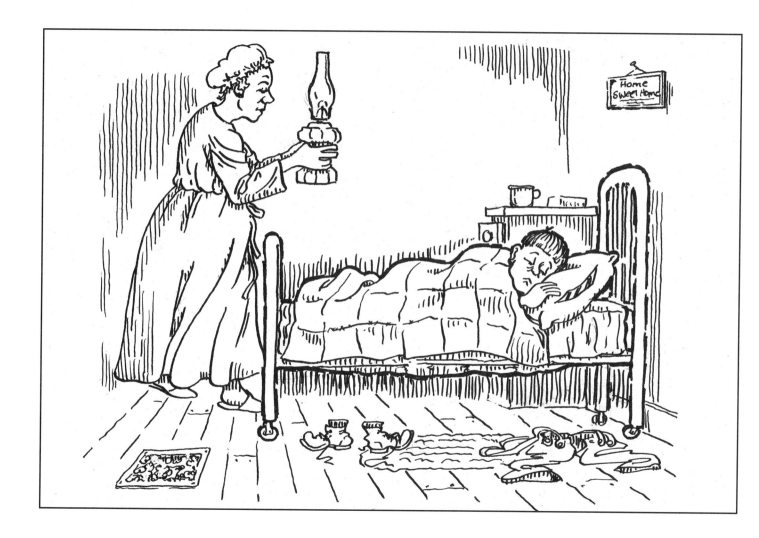

Dear Dad:

We won't forget the stories you told us when we were kids. Stories like your courtship with Mom. Sometimes you went to see her on a bike with bald tires—ten kilometers one way. You had to pass a farmer's huge dog that barked in your ear as you tried to out-peddle him. Sometimes you got three or four flat tires in one trip. You were thrilled that Mom's mother was young enough at heart to ride around on the bike while you two visited. Sometimes you rode on horseback. Once you were caught in a rainstorm coming home—your curfew was ten o'clock—and you got lost in the pitch-black night. You rode around in circles until the sun came up. Your first little farmhouse, after you married, "wasn't much to write home about," you always said. A cow or two. An outdoor toilet. Two kilometers from the closest neighbor. One Sunday coming home from church, you were upset into a snowbank from the horse-drawn cart. The big Depression of the 30s hit soon after you started out together, but you both always said those years together were great. You trusted God to help you with problems. You lived on love and faith.

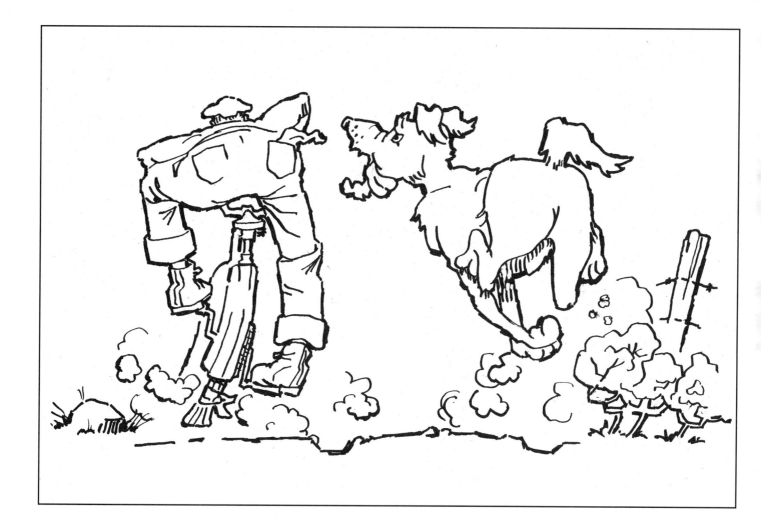

Dear Dad:

I remember how you shaved Sunday mornings before going to church. You lathered your face with white shaving cream, sharpened your razor blade back and forth on the leather strap hanging from the knob of a chair beside you, and scraped away the cream, leaving bare patches of brown, leathery skin. I remember sitting beside you in church later, sneaking *Sen Sen* mints from the little pocket inside the big pocket of your suit. You smelled sweet. But when we came home from church something changed drastically. You put on your work clothes. They had a very different smell to them—the smell of the barn. It was like having two dads—a Sunday-best dad and a work-a-day dad. I loved them both!

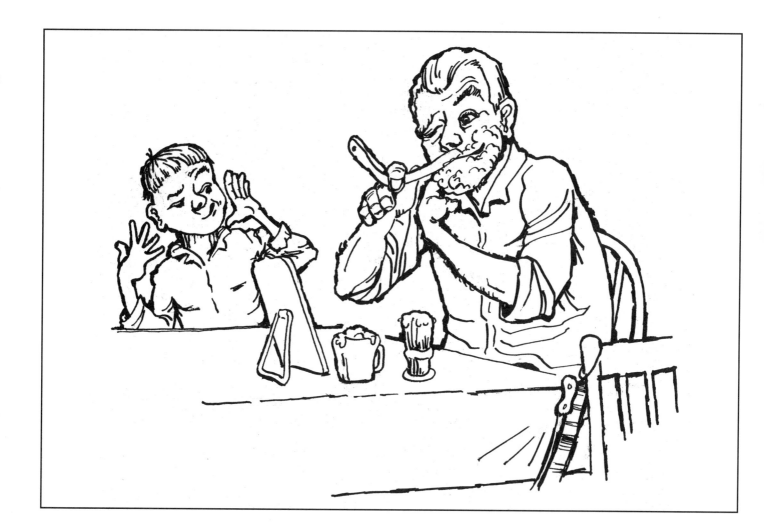

Dear Dad:

I remember postponing my bedtime on summer nights, waiting for you to come home from the fields, waiting to hear the stories of what you saw while you worked. There were the little foxes playing around their heedful mothers, always venturing a little further into their new worlds. The hawk, circling high in the sky, swooping down on a careless gopher, flying up and away to a rock and making a meal of the catch. The prairie chicken cocks in the mating season, parading their finest stuff in front of the hens. The meadowlark's nest you carefully moved out of the way of the tractor and how you watched for the mother bird to re-orient herself to the new location. You said God might ask us someday whether we ever took time to enjoy the little wonders of His creation, and we'd tell Him we were too busy working. You thought this would make Him sad.

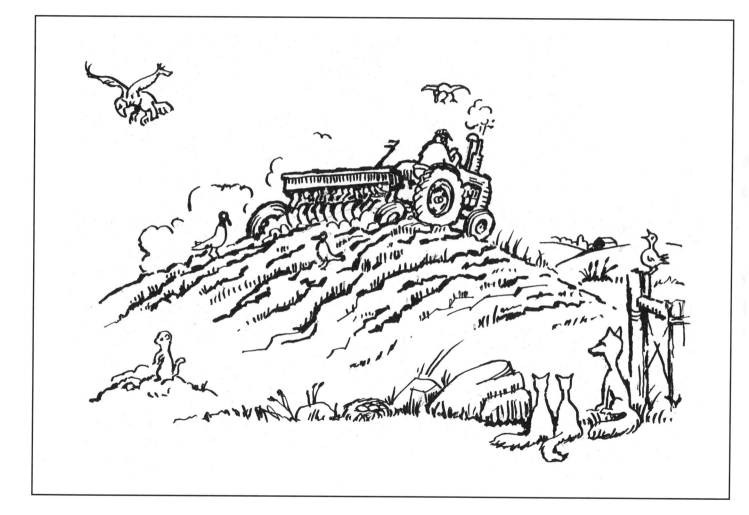

Dear Dad:

HAPPY BIRTHDAY!

Do you remember the summer evenings we cranked out homemade ice cream for birthdays? Someone had to get the ice and the cream from the icehouse, where there always seemed to be a lizard or garter snake under the straw covering the ice for insulation. We put the ice in a gunnysack and smashed it. When everything was ready we alternated turning the crank until it wouldn't turn anymore. We ate the ice cream with puffed wheat and you always teased the person who coughed first. Homemade ice cream was just one of the ways you and Mom made us feel very special. Thank-you!

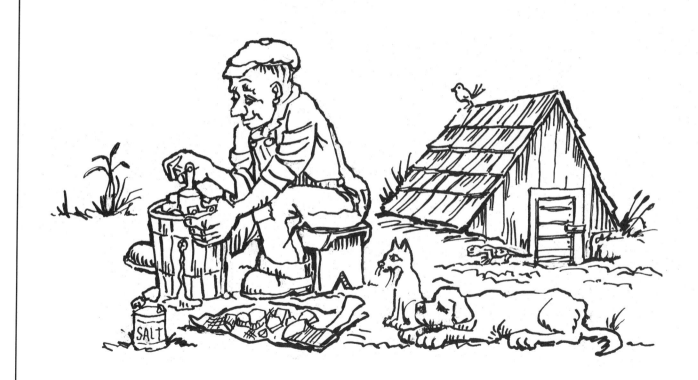

Dear Dad:

Do you remember potato-planting time in spring? You hitched the old Case tractor to the plow and made a furrow. Mom taught us to cut the potatoes so each piece had an eye. Carrying the pieces in pails, we pressed them into the soft, wet, newly ploughed dirt, and one step apart, always with the eye up. When you came round with the tractor you made a new row as you covered the first one up. How exciting it was to find the first wrinkly potato plants peeking out of the ground about two weeks later. You were a good provider, Dad, and taught us a lot about working carefully while you prayed for rain.

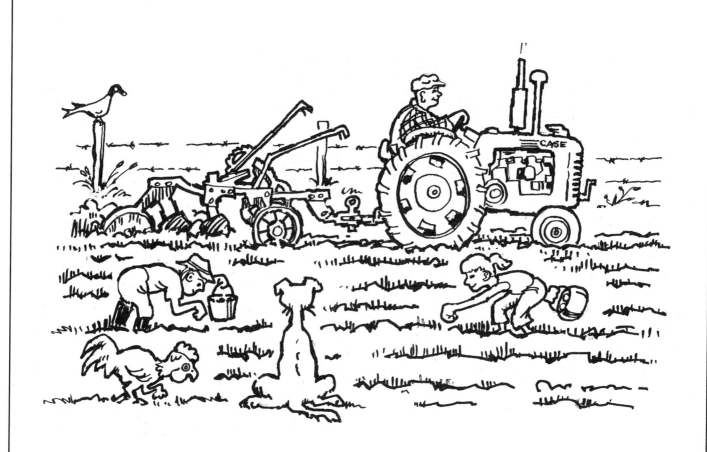

Dear Dad:

Some of my most peaceful memories are of traveling home winter evenings in the one-horse sleigh, after visiting friends in the community. The moonbeams sparkled on the snow, making the night almost as bright as day. We were wrapped in blankets, chatting family talk to the musical harmony of jingling bells, hoof beats and the squeak of the sleigh runners on the packed trail. In the daytime this trip would have been boring, and we kids would have been standing on the back runners trying to push each other off to warm up or more likely, just to be silly. But at night under the stars it was so good to sit cozily in the security of our blankets, our parents and the star-stunning world of our loving Creator.

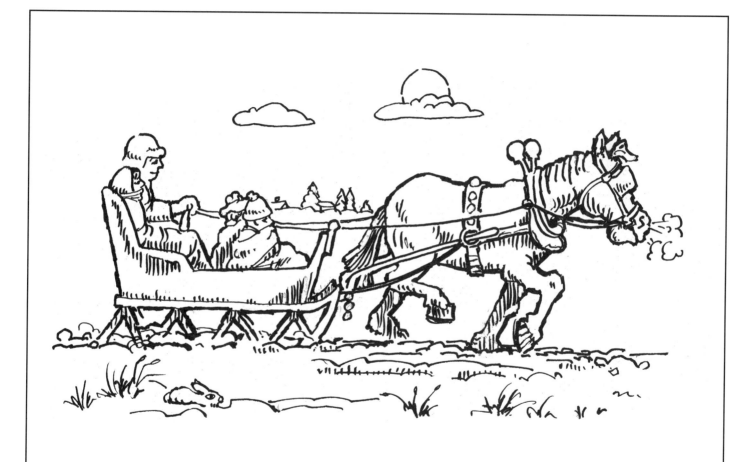

Dear Dad:

Do you remember the calls you used to make on the old country telephone, the one with the crank? I especially remember the ones you made on cold winter nights to your brother. You must have been bored, because you spent literally hours planning to build things you never got around to—like snowmobiles or machines to make your work easier. I can still hear Mom kidding you about those pie-in-the-sky inventions. Those telephones were really something, with their party lines and other neighbors free to listen in. Some people learned other languages just by eavesdropping! Our ring was three long and one short, your brother's two long and one short, and you could get the operator with one ring if you pressed the little black button on the side. Remember that? No real privacy. That's how it was. But everyone understood, and there was security in knowing, on those lonely prairie winter nights, that people were as close as three long rings and one short.

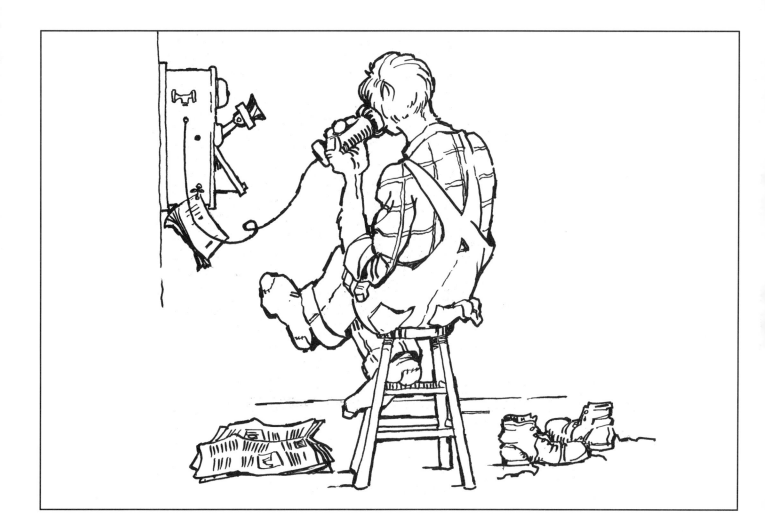

Dear Dad:

You must surely remember the Bible reading and prayer you had with us each day at breakfast. On school days it was a touch of God's presence with us before we hurried out to beat the school bell. You led us through the same ritual again each evening. That was harder to sit through. For one thing, it signaled bedtime, which we always tried to avoid as long as possible. It was also rather boring, especially your long prayer and Mom's. Kneeling for prayers, we kids often made faces at each other through the backs of our chairs, trying to make the other person laugh.

Once, years later, when you stayed at our house because you couldn't be left on your own anymore, I heard your voice in the bedroom at night. I listened at the door. You were praying. At breakfast we asked you to read from your large-print King James Bible. The corners of the pages had greasy thumbprints from your working days. You stumbled a bit, but you made it through. Now we listened closely! Your faith shone like a warm light in the farmhouse window in the night. You kept your faith till the end.

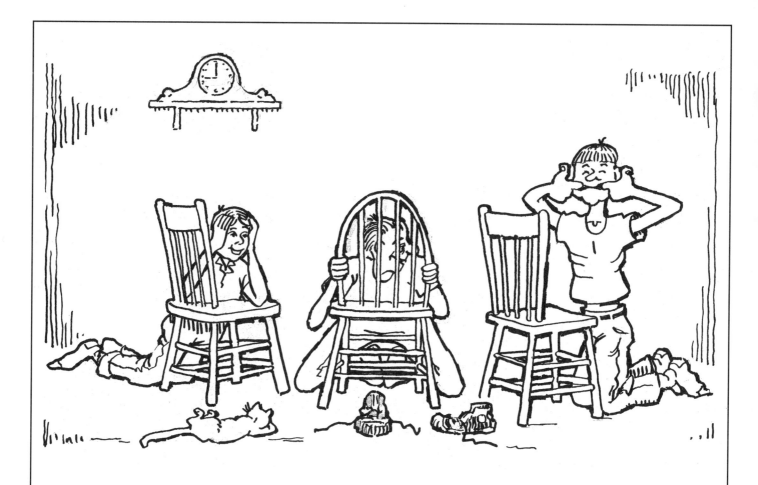

Dear Dad:

Happy Father's Day!

Do you remember the good old cow-milking days? Bossy and Blacky and Molly? And there was Amos the cat, patting your leg, begging for a squirt, with Jip the dog wanting some too, though he was more polite. Sorry for the many times you had to milk alone in the mornings, just because Mom couldn't rouse us out of bed on time. You've always been a patient and faithful father, and we love you very much!

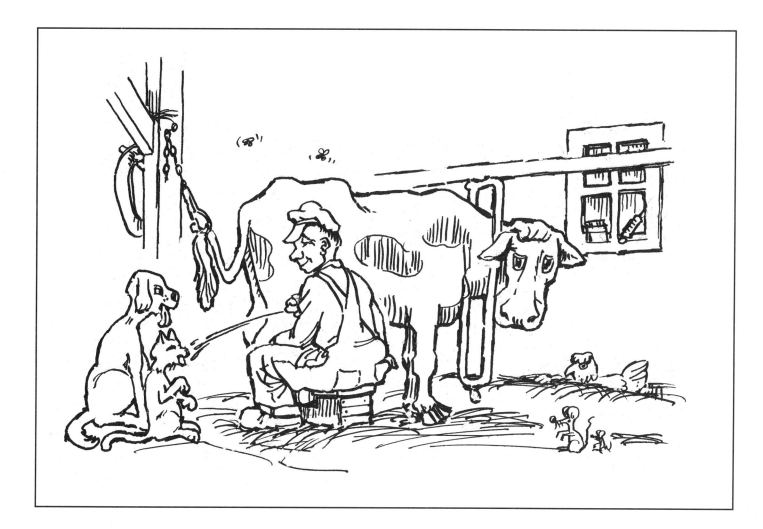

Dear Dad:

I remember when you were our church Sunday school superintendent. One of the most exciting times was Christmas when we put on a long program of plays, songs and recitations under the lights of the gas lamps. Reciting a verse in front of friends, maybe even girlfriends, was embarrassing, especially when we got older and forgot our lines. But we were never too old to enjoy the brown paper bags filled with Christmas oranges, nuts, candies and a box of Cracker Jack. We'd say our piece if that's what it took to get the treat. These performances were an excellent preparation for the future, even though we didn't realize it then. Today we thank you for your leadership in giving us those wonderful experiences.

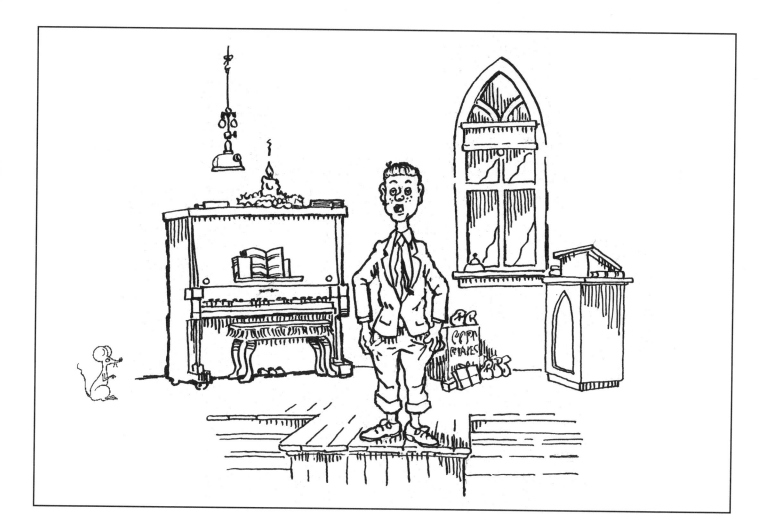

Dear Dad:

You always had to live with the wind, didn't you? You were tanned brown from working outside all day. Maybe that's why you and Mom never forgot the Dirty Thirties with the blowing dust and the tumbleweeds. You told us about those hardships often enough. But instead of complaining, you used the wind. I remember when you built the windmill to generate electricity. You designed the wooden parts and carved the propeller out of a long two-by-six plank, balancing it perfectly. I watched you and was proud of you. I think you were ahead of your time. During windstorms the family helped you worry about overcharging the sixteen glass storage batteries connected in the basement. Sometimes I get lonesome for the hum the anchor wires outside my upstairs bedroom window made on sub-zero nights. I often went to sleep to their music. Somehow they helped me feel secure. When we needed light, you saw to it that it was there.

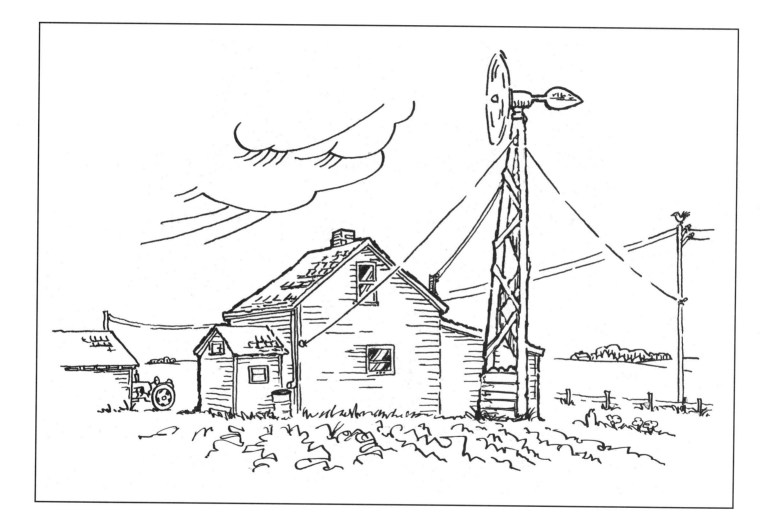

Dear Dad:

It was well after you had retired off the family farm. You still really enjoyed going out there from town to do odd jobs. On this particular day I was with you and you decided to plow up a few acres of land on the back forty. I'd forgotten how scary this job could be. Steep hills. Badger holes almost big enough to fall into. Rocks that threatened to upset the tractor backwards. I worried about your safety. But it was no problem to you. You were as relaxed as if you'd been sitting in the kitchen reading the farm paper. As I pondered this, I recognized why. It was 70 years of familiarity. Here were three old friends–the man, the land and the machine–blended into one. Familiar and very professional.

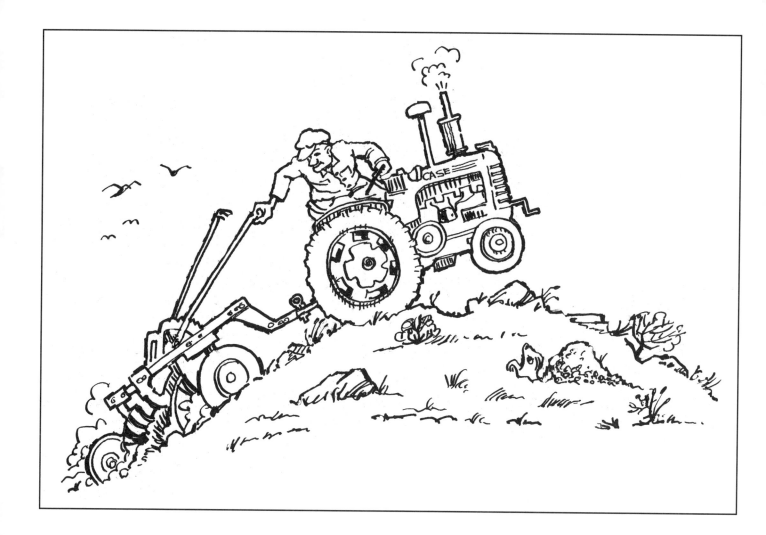

Dear Dad:

Do you remember the beautiful summer evening you and I cleared away the foundation of the old country schoolhouse? Built by the first settlers in the area, the school sat on a yard next to the land you farmed. It was the only public school you ever attended. When they moved the school away you took over the old yard, along with the task of clearing away the broken foundation. A beautiful prairie sunset was shaping up and the killdeers called to each other as their ancestors had for thousands of years. As we chained the tractor to a corner piece of concrete you discovered, to your surprise, the initials of the school's pioneer builders, drawn in the wet cement many years earlier. Your father's initials were there too and you became noticeably sentimental. Was it just my imagination, or did you move those crumbling chunks of cement with a loving touch of reverence after that?

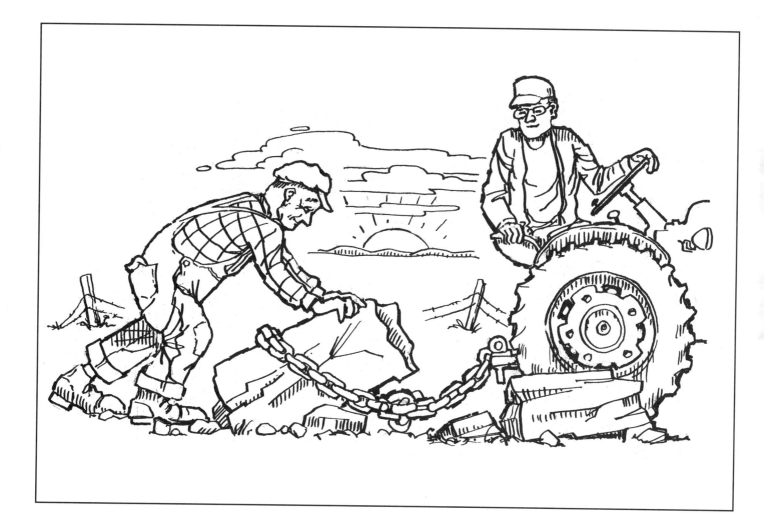

Dear Dad:

As a child I looked up to you as someone who knew what to do in every situation. I saw that begin to change one day when you were visiting us in the city and I took you for a city bus ride. At the bus stop I made sure you had the right amount of change. The bus stopped. We got on. I put my change in the fare box and went ahead to find a seat. You followed me on, but didn't know where to put the fare money. You placed it carefully on the ledge beside the slot. The driver got upset with you in front of the other passengers. He gave you a lecture about putting fares in the proper place and made you come back and do it right. I felt very badly for you. I had wanted to save your dignity by not doing for you what you could do for yourself. In the end you lost more than we saved. It was a turning point for me. I started to think of doing things for you I'd never done before. I began to ponder what our future relationship might be like.

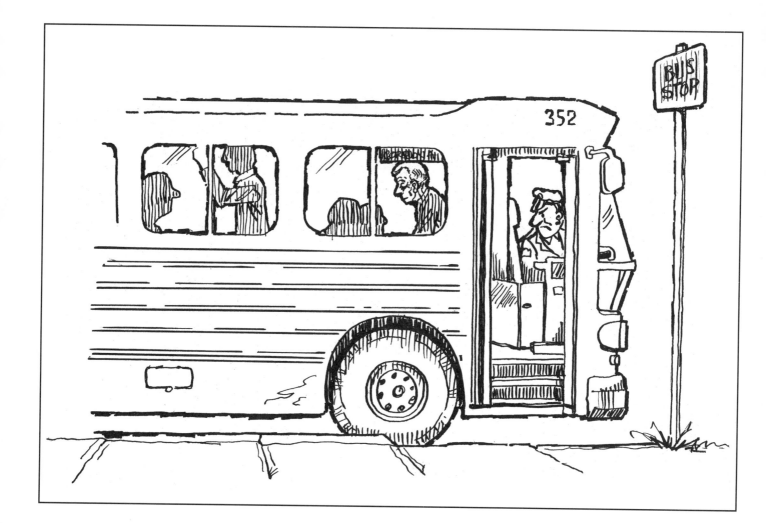

Dear Dad:

I remember clearly the painful day of Mom's surgery. For some time she had experienced difficulty swallowing. The doctor's fears that it was stomach cancer came true. Mom was cheerful in the hospital room that morning when they wheeled in the stretcher, touching her toes a couple of times and then hoisting herself up without help. The surgeon said if it was a three-hour surgery, there would be hope. If it lasted only an hour, this meant nothing further could be done. We waited fretfully. The voice on the intercom calling the family to Mom's room came exactly an hour later. After the surgeon gently explained to us that she might have three more months to live, I watched you study her quiet, unconscious form and the tubing supporting her. You held her unresponsive hand for a long, long time. Finally you sighed and said, "Well, we've been through this before." You recalled Mom's mother who also died of cancer, and your brother-in-law and your own father. There must be something about remembering the past journey of life's experiences that helps us cope. God carried you in those times and you knew He would carry all of us again.

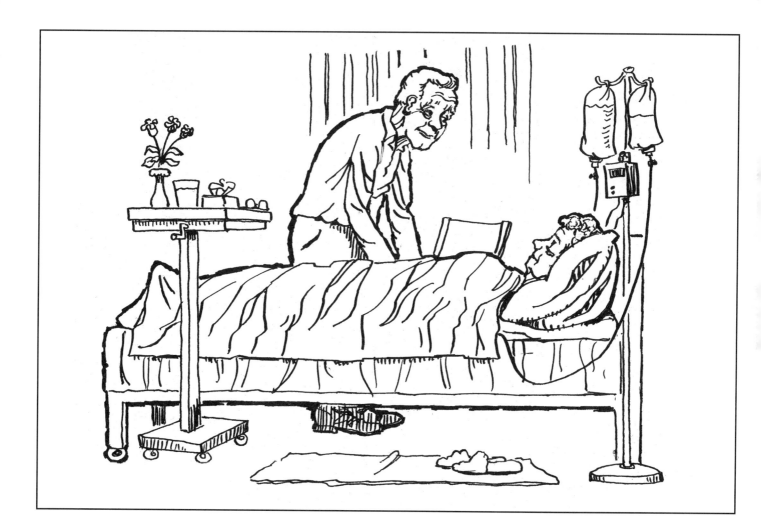

Dear Dad:

You were very anxious about Mom's gravestone. Do you remember how important it was to you? You checked prices. You visited cemeteries to find out what you liked. You didn't want to do it alone, however, and finally we decided together. You picked the verse, "EVER LOVED, EVER REMEMBERED." There was no doubt in your mind that it should be a double headstone, for both of you. Thinking of all the flowers and crafts she made for family and friends, you chose the symbol of roses for Mom. For yourself you chose heads of wheat, so very appropriate for a man of the soil. When the stone was installed we went to view it at the cemetery. I'll always remember how you stood there against the sunset. Your voice broke when you said, "Someday we'll be here together and she'll be lying at my right side, next to my heart."

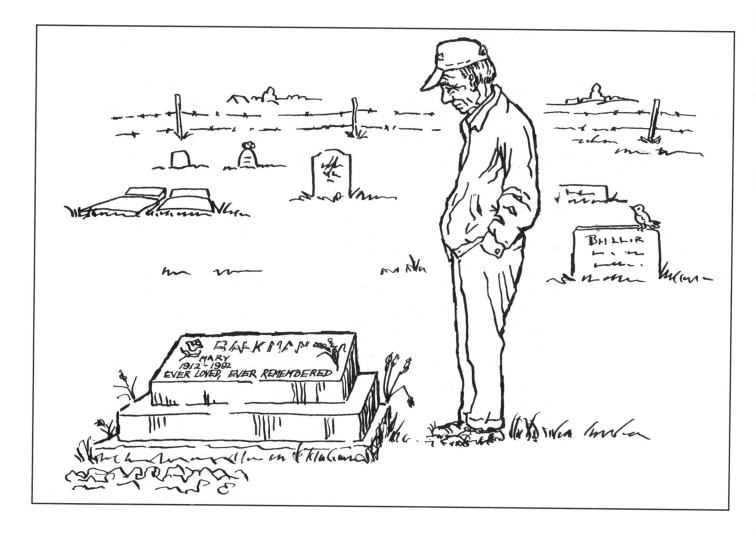

Dear Dad:

Since Mom is gone, we'll probably never know what went on between the two of you as your memory began to fade. We saw her get impatient with you when you didn't catch on to things, but then it was easy to blame it on your hearing aid. She probably covered for you because she didn't want you to be embarrassed, or maybe she couldn't herself admit what was happening. After all, she knew there were people in your family line who had lost their memory too. Perhaps she was trying to tell us something when she recounted the night the two of you were coming home and you drove into the wrong town and insisted it was home. She never did say how you got out of there. She did let on there was an argument. We began to notice you became disoriented more easily in the evening, in the dark. And that's about the time she died. Was she spared a lot of pain? We know she was very committed to you. "In sickness and in health," you promised each other at your wedding. We know she would have done all she could.

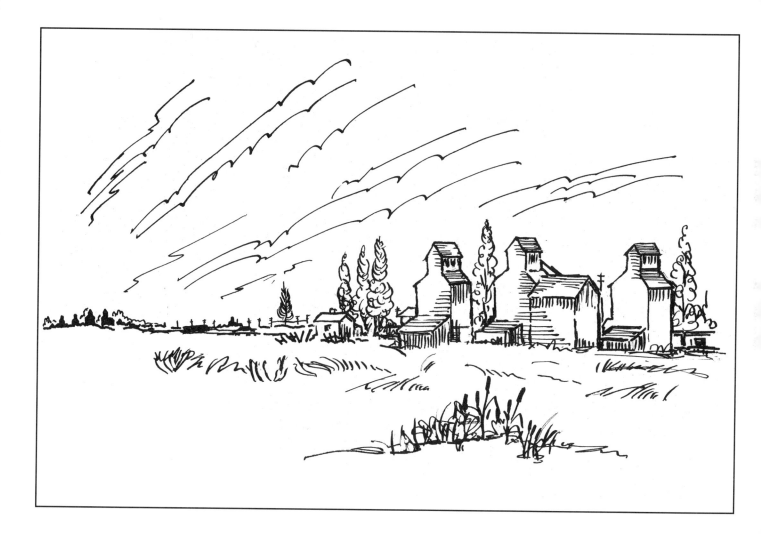

Dear Dad:

It was funny and sad at the same time. You had started painting your house alone one summer. The neighbors were concerned as they watched you high up on the ladder, but they couldn't persuade you to wait until family came. You were "on a roll." I came to help, starting by painting the patches you missed. You kept losing your paintbrush. You'd disappear to the back of the house and come back after a long time scratching your head. You forgot what you went there for, you said. We laughed about it together and got you all fixed up with your brush to go on painting again. When this happened a second time, it troubled me. What was going on?

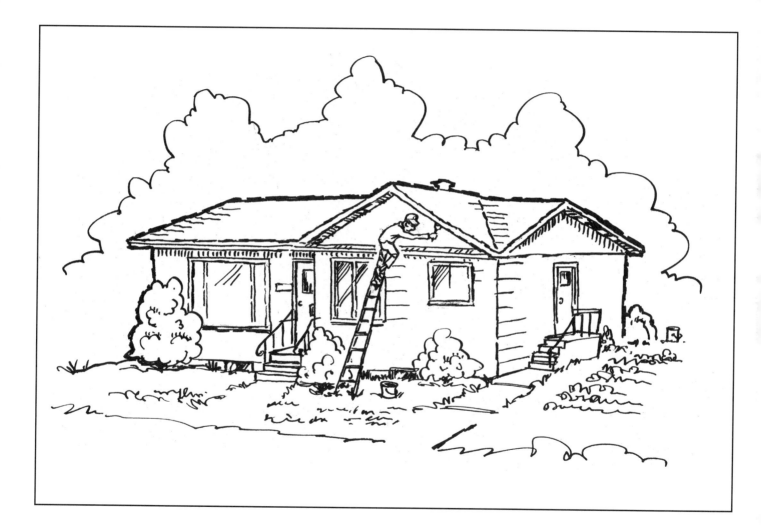

Dear Dad:

Do you remember how you learned to cook after Mom died? You learned to make breakfast–porridge, eggs and toast–earlier when Mom had surgery. But now you had to make two more meals a day. Boiled potatoes were easiest and you worked with the meat Mom had canned or left in the freezer, and pickles. The day we painted your house you decided to bake an apple pie a neighbor lady had brought over for your freezer. You set the oven temperature carefully, but insisted a baking pie had to be watched to get it just right. I came in from painting to check how you were doing and whether you could still handle the stove safely. I found you peering into the oven every few minutes. You couldn't find the oven light switch, so you used the greasy yellow trouble light from your shop downstairs. Well, why not? After all, you used it to fix all those car motors over the years. You wanted to learn to cook, you said, and you really got to enjoy it. You taught us how much people can learn after 80.

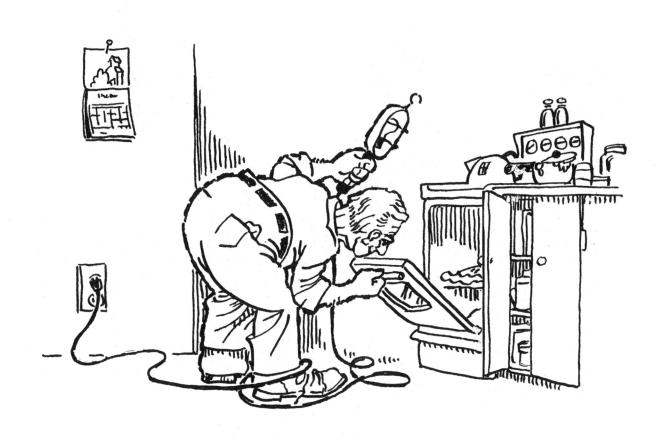

Dear Dad:

I remember when we found evidence you were wandering around the house at night. You had trouble finding the bathroom, though it was next to your bedroom. We were afraid you might even go outside and get lost in the dark. One night when I stayed with you I turned on a night light so you could find your way around. I even barricaded the hallway with furniture so you couldn't miss the bathroom door and wander away. I was pleased, in the morning, to see it had worked! The barricade was in place, just as it had been left the night before. It was only when I stepped out the back door into the morning sunlight that I had a shocking surprise. There in the snow were the unmistakable prints of your bare feet.

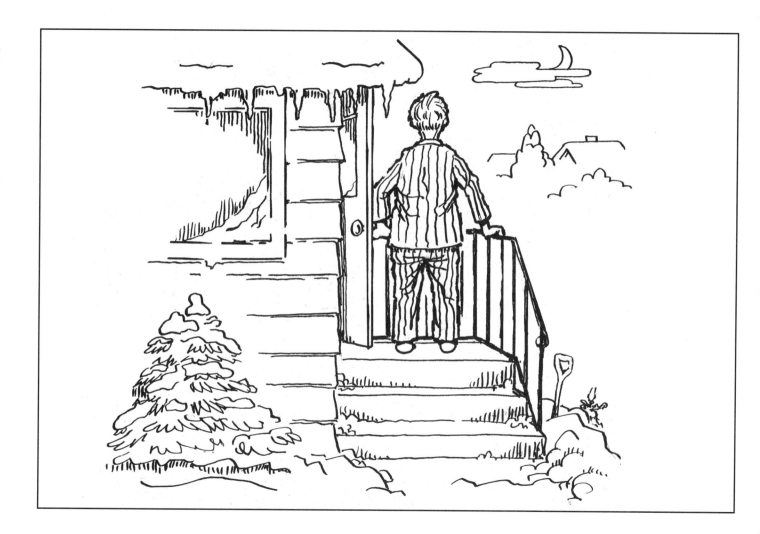

Dear Dad:

It was hard to see your memory slip away. It was even harder to take over things you'd always looked after so well all your life. Like your checkbook. At first you kept paying your bills yourself, while we kept an eye on your checkbook entries. The family agreed that I should be the one to help you with your finances. We explained the situation at your local bank. They were very helpful. When you started losing track and forgot to write in the entries, I wrote them in for you. Once when I came to visit, you were very upset! You were planning to call a family meeting about me. My handwriting in your record book was confusing you. You were convinced I was writing checks behind your back—stealing, you called it—and you were very serious about telling the rest of the family so! They all understood. But it hurt anyways. For a whole day you treated me with suspicion. Eventually you forgot and then it wasn't a problem any more.

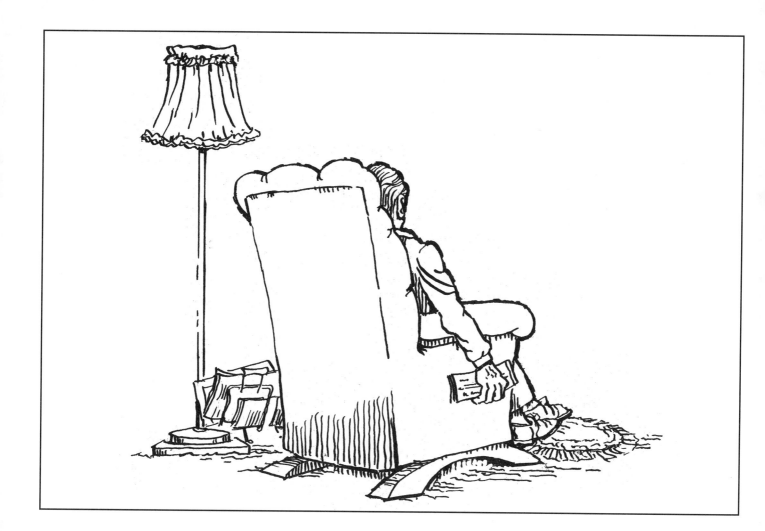

Dear Dad:

I wish we could have avoided the weekend we sold your car. You still owned the house in town and we took you out of the personal care home for the day. You knew something was going on, but you couldn't remember the details we patiently repeated to you. In the afternoon you came to me, held out your hand and said firmly, "I want the keys!" How things had changed since I was a teenager asking you for the keys. We went out to the garage. You got in behind the steering wheel and I sat beside you. You started the motor, listened lovingly and critically, the way you always did to every vehicle you owned. You turned it off, tried it again, tried the signals, the wipers, the horn and the lights. You noticed that the muffler was leaking. Then you turned the engine off for the very last time and we went back into the house. You tried to be stoical, but I knew you were grieving inside. Two weeks later the driver's license you had held for 60 years quietly expired.

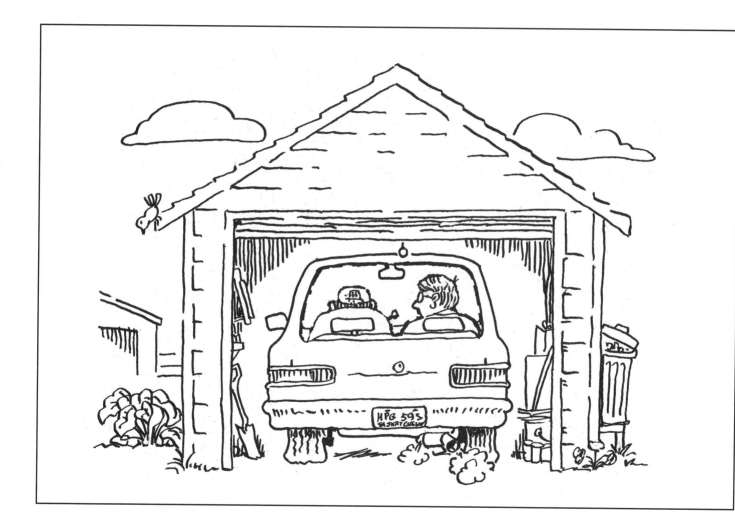

Dear Dad:

Do you remember those rare times when you coyly strung us kids along about the first time you and Mom kissed, somewhere out in Grandpa's cow pasture? You enjoyed teasing Mom about it until she blushed and then you'd chuckle, without ever telling us the rest of the story. After Mom was gone and we saw that living alone was too difficult for you, one of your grandsons stayed in your house with you at night. One evening you came into his bedroom to talk. You were drawn to your black and white wedding picture hanging on the wall and made some endearing comments about Mom. The next day your grandson saw you in the room again, alone, holding the picture. After you left, he noticed a smudge on the glass of the picture. Looking more closely, he recognized the imprint of your lips on Mom in her wedding gown. We never told you, but when the rest of your grandchildren came to visit, they all took their turn checking the glass for that smudge of love. I guess that's as close as we'll ever come to the little secret you and Mom shared about your first kiss in Grandpa's cow pasture.

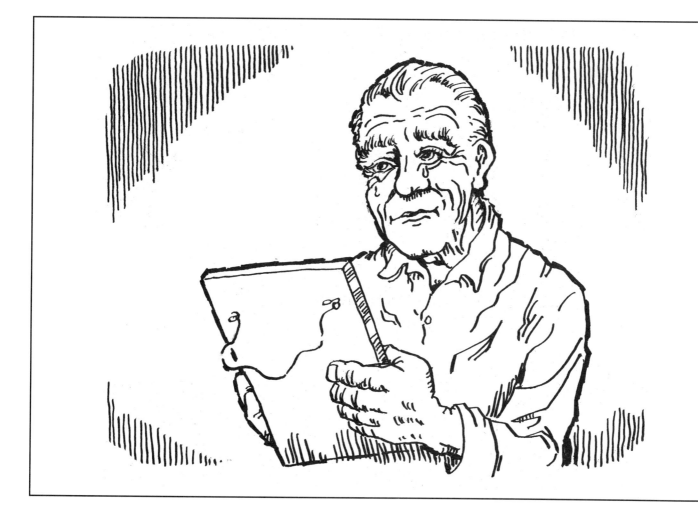

Dear Dad:

Very graciously you agreed that it had to be done. But your body language betrayed your mixed feelings. It was the Christmas after Mom died and we had to start cleaning up the things she left behind. Instead of picking names for a Christmas box that year, the grandchildren were invited to choose keepsakes for themselves. If two or more wanted the same item, they had to do their own negotiating. It was like a big free garage sale—old magazines, jewelry, craft projects, ornaments, windup toys, Rogers Golden Syrup pails and most special of all, the "gramma blankets" made by Gramma herself from old cloth remnants she had patiently cut into squares and sewn together. You sat on a recliner in the middle of it all and watched. For a while you looked genuinely amused remembering Mom and proud of how her handiwork was being cherished. In the excitement we almost missed the distant look that came into your eyes and the trace of a tear in each corner. Was it sadness that came with missing Mom? Or was it thankfulness at seeing her loving spirit passed on to the next generation? Maybe both!

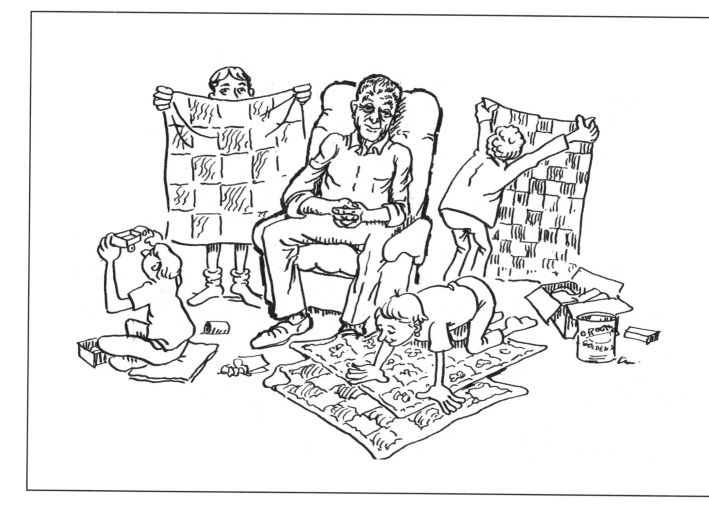

Dear Dad:

I remember phoning you right after you were admitted into the care home. They called you to the phone at the nursing station. First you described how they gave you the important job of helping people in their wheelchairs. Then you lowered your voice so no one else could hear. You wanted to know what I thought about them sewing nametags on all your clothes. You didn't trust them. You seemed to think it was an invasion of your privacy. You also begged for some money. You said you were embarrassed not to have cash on you in case you needed to buy something. I hung up the phone with a deep sadness, feeling like a conniver in these indignities. Things that you had always controlled were being taken away from you and you were sensing the losses very keenly.

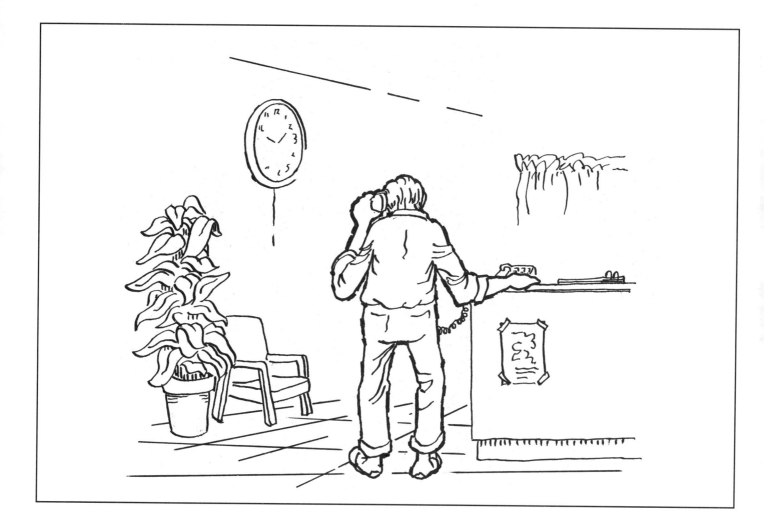

Dear Dad:

Do you remember the Christmas you bought us kids an electric train? The crops must have been good that year. We had begged for years and you were always sympathetic, maybe because of the fascination you had with steam locomotives and diesel engines yourself. Sometimes you wished out loud that you could have trained to be a diesel mechanic, but you never had the opportunity. That Christmas Eve, our ears to the kitchen door, we heard you playing with something that sounded very exciting. When we tore the wrapper off the box the next day, there was the train! The excitement was almost too much. You seemed never to lose your fascination for machines. Maybe that's why one of the nurses in the care home had to run after you and get you off the railway tracks when you sneaked out to watch a freight train speed through town. Some longings do not leave us.

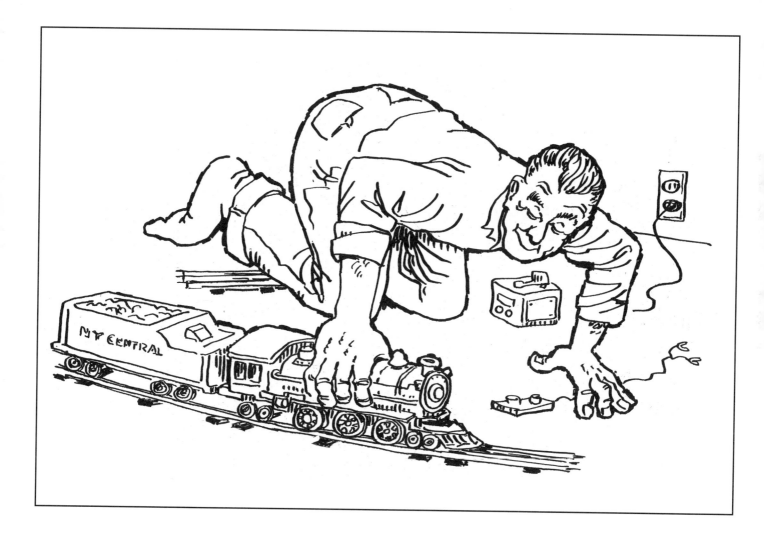

Dear Dad:

I still feel guilty that we didn't take you along to the wedding of your first grandchild. The two of you had spent a lot of time together as he was growing up. You taught him about machines. Maybe that's why he became a mechanical engineer. He wanted very much for you to be there, but you were living in the personal care home, really quite disoriented. You were healthy, mobile and still a handsome old gentleman, but we thought you'd get upset about something or be loud, and that you'd be disoriented staying in a new place. I explained that we were going out of town to the wedding and should I take a message along from you? You had learned to cover yourself quite well and I'm not sure you were really aware of what I was asking, but you did say, "Well. . . wish them a happy life together." Were we being too easy on ourselves? Would you have managed better than we thought because you'd be with family? We'll never know. It was hard to drive away from you, standing alone in the home lounge with that pleading look on your face.

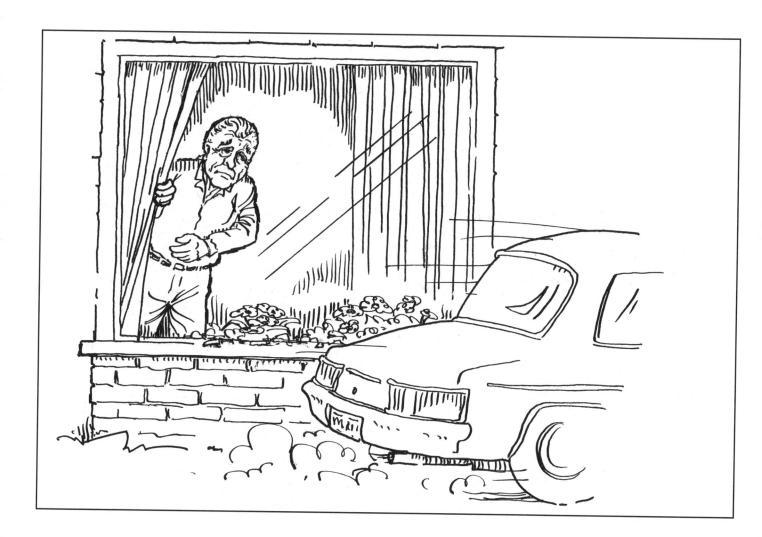

Dear Dad:

Your favorite hymn was "My Jesus I Love Thee." You requested it most in the little country church we attended. You boomed it out on the battered old bass horn you played in the church band, and sometimes you sang it around the house. Your singing and whistling were always reassuring. When Mom's cancer struck, and while you tried your best to look after her, you sang even more. You never seemed to forget those hymns, even when you had to move into the personal care home. The nurses told us that as you lost track of time you kept your roommate awake in the middle of the night by singing to him. They put you in the chapel, gently shut the door and let you sing to your heart's content, "My Jesus, I love Thee, I know Thou art mine."

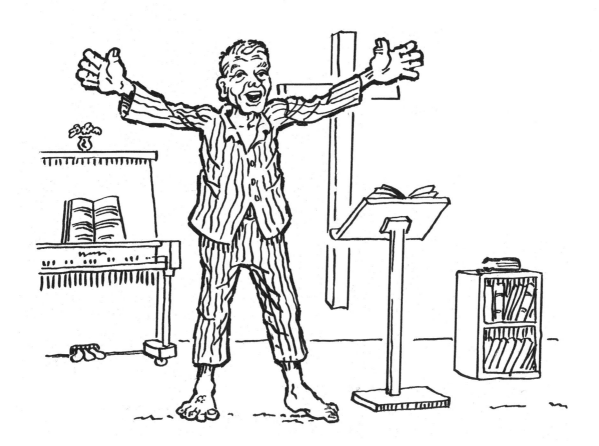

Dear Dad:

You probably don't remember the day we took you out of the personal care home to plant potatoes. As usual, you were disoriented. We hadn't sold your house yet, so we decided to plant potatoes in the spot where Mom had maintained her lush garden. The shadows of your mind lifted for a while that afternoon and you acted much like you used to, only a bit slower. You helped cut the seed potatoes, lecturing us on how each piece had to be cut so it had an eye. You felt in charge again as you told us how to plant them. Eye up. Not too deep. Step hard on each spot. Not too fast! Don't get careless! You obviously relished the responsibility and it seemed you wanted this project to go on for as long as possible. A month later we brought you back to the garden. The plants were up. You remembered putting in the seeds. You made a close inspection of each plant for potato bugs. You knocked them off with a vengeance! This turned out like the community health care nurse had said. Watch for the short moments when the shadows lift and treasure them. We did.

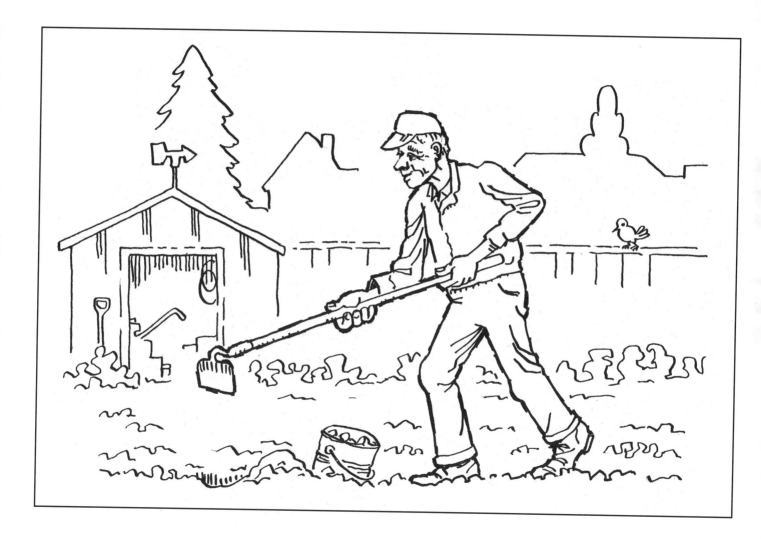

Dear Dad:

You always enjoyed fishing. You and your buddies would go out to your little pond in the hills and have a good time together. You took one of your granddaughters out and taught her to fish. I know she'll never forget that. But the time came when you didn't go fishing anymore. You were having trouble remembering how to get there and your friends weren't comfortable taking you. When you moved into the personal care home and we saw you getting bored, we brought you one of your old fishing reels. You spent hours in your room taking it apart and putting it together. Over and over again like a child exploring a new toy. We wondered what was going through your mind. Did you think you were at the old fishing spot? Were you remembering the feel of a good catch? Did you think you were going out again? We had no way of finding out. So many things in your life turned around when you began to lose memory.

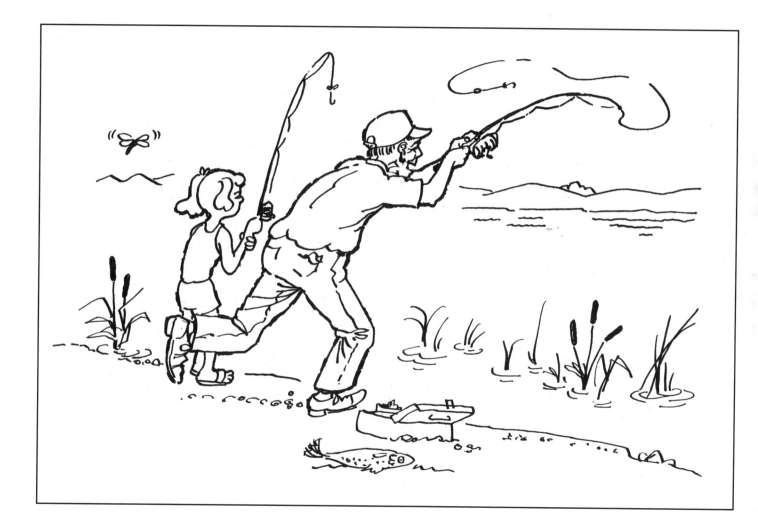

Dear Dad:

I remember watching you cut your father's hair. You cut mine too–many, many times–and eventually you taught me to cut yours. It was always a close, personal time with relaxed, easy conversations. I remember sweeping up the clippings. Mine were black and yours had become white. I recall standing there reflecting that someday mine would be white too. I still think about the last haircut I gave you. Your mind was wandering and you talked nonsensically about things from the past. Halfway through you became silent. In one of those moments when the curtains of your mind opened briefly, you said that one of these days this would be your last haircut and then Mom wouldn't be in heaven alone. Then you went back to rambling again. I wondered what you were trying to tell me. It was the last haircut I gave you. A month later you were taken to the hospital.

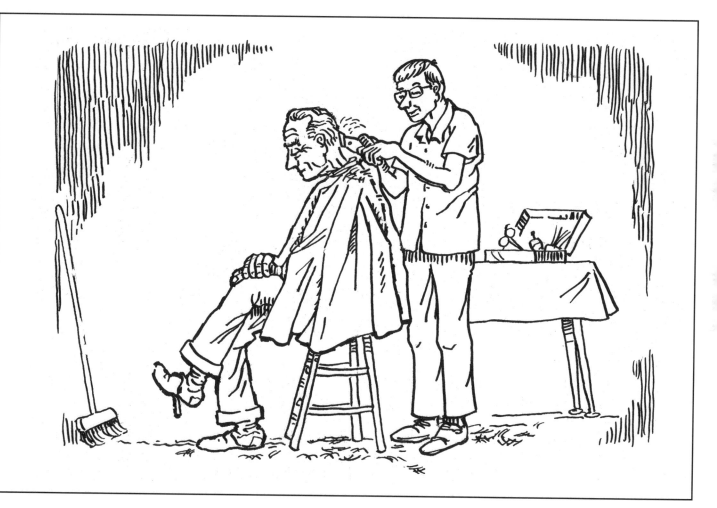

Dear Dad:

Your family remembers one of the last times we brought you from the personal care home to your house. Most of your grandchildren were there. When Mom died we opened her old trunk full of precious things she'd saved over the years. Her wedding dress was there, neatly folded, along with the wax flowers, crushed now. There was a box with the beads she wore and the pressed handkerchief you wore in your suit pocket. We peeked under a cardboard liner and found a yellow envelope. It was a love letter you wrote Mom the winter before you were married. It was postmarked "Flowing Well, Jan. 1, 1933." That was the name of the place where you lived, but in the letter you wrote it as "Flowing Love." One of the grandchildren read it aloud to the rest of us. You spoke about your love for Mom and then signed it, "Your lonesome Sweetheart." Now, 60 years later, we knew you still missed her and would want to have her close to you. Before dinner we asked you to pray, just as you had many times before. You prayed slowly, struggling to remember, for your family, thankful to God for His love and care. When you said "Amen", there wasn't a dry eye in the house.

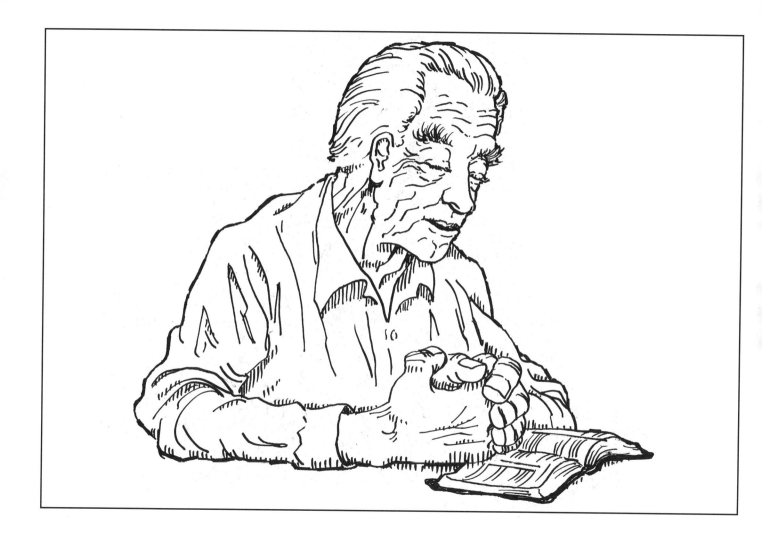

Dear Dad:

I'll never forget the last goodbye we said to each other. It was a few days before our daughter's wedding. They said you were forgetting to swallow and that you were very sick. I caught an overnight bus and walked from the depot to the hospital. I had tried to prepare myself by praying and reading Psalms from the Bible. The nurse at the desk was surprised to see me and asked if I was prepared for the visit. I said, "Yes," and she took me into your room. You'd been unconscious all night, but now you stirred when I talked to you. I took your large, weak hand in mine and you moved it around to let me know you knew I was there. You tried hard to say something. But couldn't. The look in your eyes was more loving than anything I'd ever seen from you before. I prayed with you and sang, "My Jesus I Love Thee," and then read a letter from one of your granddaughters. Your breathing got slower and slower. Finally it stopped. I sat beside the bed for a long time, holding your hand, going through memories and wondering what it was like for you, now in heaven. Finally you could see the One you sang about so often in the song, "My Jesus I Love Thee."

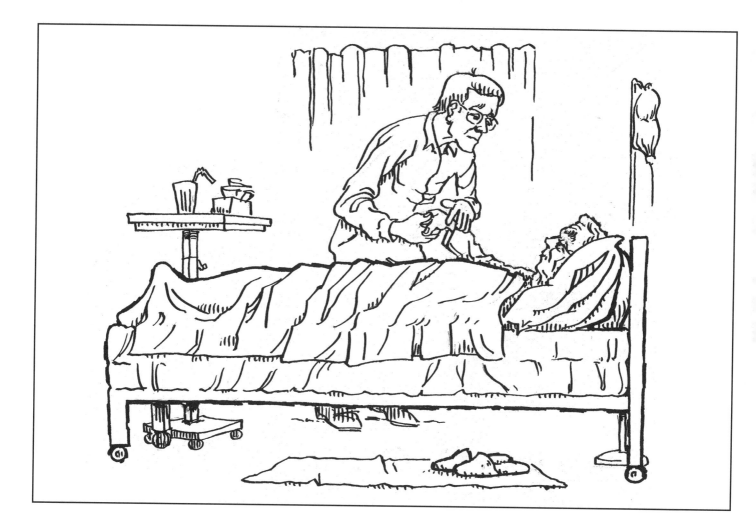

Dear Dad:

I don't really have to tell you this. You and Mom may have seen it all from your balcony vantage point in heaven. The funeral was beautiful—a celebration of life. Beside the casket we had a table with some of your treasures: tools, songbooks, your Bible, the old fishing reel. The pastor you and Mom always appreciated so much helped us cry, but also directed us to God for hope and gratitude. Your grandchildren carried the casket from the hearse into the little country church cemetery at sunset. I'll never forget the lonely sound of the flute as your niece played "My Jesus I Love Thee." We buried you beside Mom at the gravestone you so carefully chose for her a few years earlier. And then we said our last goodbye, till we meet again, in heaven.

Ever loved, ever remembered.

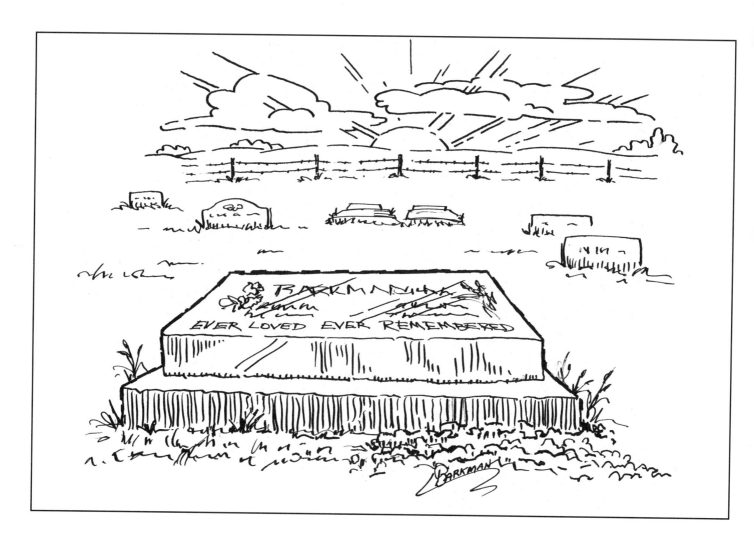

About the Author

A gifted communicator, Lorlie has found that he can be most effective by talking with words and pictures, drawing out people with visual storytelling. After studying commercial art by correspondence, his ambition was to be an editorial cartoonist, which he pursued briefly with the *Swift Current Sun*, in Saskatchewan where he was born and raised. His cartoons have been published in the *Mennonite Brethren Herald*, *The Christian Leader* and *Christianity Today*. Lorlie is currently free-lancing in ministry and communication.

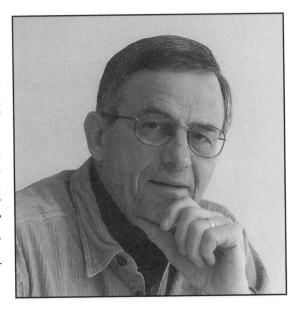

Lorlie has pastored churches for 19 years in Moose Jaw, Saskatchewan and Winnipeg, Manitoba. For 15 years he was the producer of *The Third Story*, a children's television series produced at Mennonite Bretheren Communications in Winnipeg. He is a graduate of Bethany Bible Institute and Mennonite Brethren Bible College (Concord College).

Lorlie and his wife Deanna are beginners at grandparenting. They have three married children.